THE ULTIMATE METABOLIC RESET EXERCISE FOR WOMEN

With Powerful Exercises to Increase Metabolism, Long-Term Weight Loss, Flexibility, and Fitness Improvement, You Can Discover Your Body's Potential.

Vincent John Walker

DISCLAIMER

This publication is designed to provide competent and reliable information regarding the subject covered. However, the views expressed in this publication are those of the author alone, and should not be taken as expert instruction or professional advice. The reader is responsible for his or her actions. The author hereby disclaims any responsibility or liability whatsoever that is incurred from the use or application of the contents of this publication by the purchaser of the reader. The purchaser or reader is hereby responsible for his or her actions.

Table of Contents

INTRODUCTION

The Ultimate Metabolic Reset Exercise Program for Women is the start of an incredible journey that will completely transform your perspective on exercise and wellness. In a world where the stresses of modern life often leave us feeling listless and disconnected from our bodies, this program is a breath of fresh air. Examining the relationship between exercise, energy, and metabolism, takes a more comprehensive approach than just going to the gym and putting in some miles on the treadmill.

Imagine waking up every morning feeling rejuvenated and ready to take on the world. Your body now functions like a well-oiled machine, burning fat even while you sleep and converting food into energy. This is the result of doing MRE; it's not wishful thinking.

The program's extensive understanding of the human body and its operations is one of its main selling points. The goal is to ignite your metabolism so that all of your activities contribute to your weight loss. Everything has been thoughtfully designed to support you in achieving your fitness objectives, from strength training to enhance your body's tone and form to high-intensity interval training to boost your calorie burn.

The metabolic reset workout regimen, however, addresses more than just physical well-being. The thoughtful techniques weaved throughout every session will help you not only lose weight but also feel less stressed and have more mental clarity. This is a journey that will transform your whole way of life—not it's just about becoming in shape.

Join us on an adventure that will permanently alter the way you see exercising. Imagine overcoming obstacles and embracing the self-assurance that comes from having your body and mind in harmony. The Metabolic Reset Exercise Program is a novel approach to leading a busy, fulfilling life—not it's just another workout.

Is it time to make a fresh start, rev up your metabolism, rekindle your passion for working out, and change your way of living? This is the start of an exciting journey full of possibilities. Welcome to a world where you are more than just a participant—you are the protagonist of your own story of personal development.

PHASE OF FOUNDATION: LIGHTING THE SPARK

Identifying Your Fitness Objectives

- Reflection: Consider your objectives, lifestyle, and current amount of activity. Consider why these goals are significant to you and how they relate to your overall goals.

- Setting priorities: Ascertain which of the most important goals will have the most impact on your general well-being. Concentrate on a reasonable amount of goals to prevent overburden.

- SMART Goal Setting: Make use of the following characteristics while creating your goals: time-bound, relevant, measurable, and specified.

- Make a note of them: Writing down your goals can help you stay accountable and dedicated. Remind yourself of your goals by keeping them clear.

- Divide your goals: Break larger goals down into more manageable benchmarks. Reaching these objectives makes you feel successful and keeps you inspired.

- Monitor Your Development: Regularly assess your level of development. Depending on how you're going and whatever fresh insights you've gained, modify your targets accordingly.

Metabolic Evaluation: Understanding Your Beginning Point

Crucial Elements of Metabolic Assessment:

The amount of calories your body burns when at rest is known as your resting metabolic rate, or RMR. It is the energy required to maintain basic biological processes like blood circulation and breathing. Your daily caloric needs may be calculated more easily if you know your RMR.

Analysis of Body Composition: It's important to know how much muscle there is versus fat in your body. Your visceral fat, body fat percentage, and lean muscle mass are all determined by this test. It gives you a more complete view of your health than a weight check alone.

Evaluation of Your Fitness Level: Finding areas in your training plan that could need more focus is made easier by taking a close look at your strength, flexibility, cardiovascular endurance, and other fitness components.

Health Screening: Before creating a safe and effective workout program, it is important to determine any underlying health issues, limitations, or injuries.

The Benefits of Metabolic Analysis

- Personalized Approach: You may tailor your exercise and nutrition program to your unique metabolic profile based on the results of the evaluation, ensuring that you make the most progress possible.

- Creating realistic goals: By knowing where you are today and what you want to achieve, you may set reasonable goals based on your baseline.

- Progress Monitoring: You may evaluate your progress over time and make sure you're on the right track by regularly reevaluating your performance using the same criteria.

- Prevention and Safety: You may exercise safely and make informed fitness decisions by being aware of any health hazards or limits.

Method for Metabolic Assessment:

- Professional Evaluation: A qualified fitness specialist, dietitian, or medical doctor should do the assessment. They will use specialized tools and equipment to get accurate data.

- Testing Procedures: Metabolic assessments may make use of indirect calorimetry, which evaluates carbon dioxide production and oxygen consumption, body composition scans, which employ technologies like DEXA or bioelectrical impedance, and fitness testing.

- Discussion and Analysis: As soon as you get the results, talk about them with your fitness specialist. They can help you analyze the information and build a comprehensive plan.

- Ongoing Evaluation: Arrange regular evaluations, maybe every few months, to track progress and make necessary program adjustments.

Making a Customized Exercise Program

- Goal Alignment: First Things First, your fitness goals should be supported by your training regimen. Your goals—whether they be increased cardiovascular health, weight loss, muscular development, or overall fitness—will determine which exercises are best for you.

- Exercise Selection: To provide a well-rounded approach, use a variety of exercises that concentrate on different muscle groups and fitness aspects. This may include weight training, flexibility training, cardiovascular exercises, and other activities.

- Determine the frequency of your weekly workout sessions. This might vary based on your fitness level and schedule. Rest and activity days must be balanced for optimal recovery.

- Intensity: To keep your body guessing and prevent plateaus, vary the intensity of your workouts. Include workouts of high and moderate intensity.

- Increase the weight, repetitions, or length of certain exercises to gradually increase the intensity of your workouts.

- Incorporate warm-up exercises to prepare your body for activity and cool-down exercises to enhance flexibility and recovery.

- Rest and recovery: Plan days for active recovery or rest to allow your body to heal and replenish.

How to Create a Personal Training Program

- Exam Analysis: Using the data from your fitness level assessment and metabolic analysis, ascertain your starting position and any limitations.

- Sort your objectives into priority lists by giving the various actions that will help you reach your goals a higher priority.

- Exercise Variation: Choose exercises that concentrate on different muscle groups and fitness-related topics. Exercises for the heart and lungs, muscles, flexibility, and other areas may be included in this.

- Weekly Schedule: Choose the days you'll concentrate on different training techniques and the number of days you'll exercise each week. Consider factors such as your recuperation needs and schedule.

- Exercise Sequence: Arrange exercises in a sensible order. For example, warm-up, strength training, and stretching as a cool-down should come first.

- Develop a plan for progressively increasing the level of difficulty or intensity of your exercises.

- Rest and Recovery: To help your body heal and prevent overtraining, schedule some days off or light activity.

- Flexibility: Adjust your plans as needed. Life might throw you curveballs, so be prepared to adjust your plans as needed.

- Suggestions: If you're new to working out or need guidance, consider seeing a fitness professional or using trustworthy online resources to help you create a well-rounded plan.

Fueling Your Body: Diet to Accelerate Metabolism

To improve your metabolic efficiency and get the most out of your workouts during the Metabolic Reset Exercise program, nutrition is essential. Since food serves as fuel for your body, making the right dietary choices may improve your overall health, promote healing, and increase your energy levels.

Important Dietary Guidelines for Increasing Metabolic Rate:

- Beginning with balanced macronutrients: Consume a diet rich in a range of macronutrients, such as carbohydrates, proteins, and fats, to provide your body the energy it needs to function during physical activity and recover afterward.

- Meals like lean proteins, whole grains, vegetables high in fiber, and healthy fats will naturally speed up your metabolism. These are examples of foods that boost metabolism.

- Hydrolysis: Make sure you get enough fluids. Water is essential for several metabolic processes and helps maintain steady energy levels during exercise.

- Nutrition before activity: Eat a little meal or snack to provide your body access to energy before engaging in strenuous exercise. Use a mix of protein and carbs for sustained energy.

- Post-Workout Nutrition: To support muscle repair and replenish glycogen stores, eat a meal or snack rich in protein and carbohydrates after working out.

- Healthy Snacking: Select nutrient-dense snacks to prevent energy dips and maintain stable blood sugar levels throughout the day.

- Portion Control: Be mindful of serving sizes to avoid overindulging and to regulate your caloric intake in line with your goals.

Creating a Dietary Strategy:

- Caloric Needs: Calculate your daily calorie requirements based on your metabolism, level of activity, and goals. You may see a qualified dietician or use internet calculators to ascertain your requirements.

- Macro Ratios: Select a distribution of macronutrients that will assist you in reaching your goals. For instance, increasing your protein intake could aid in muscle development and recovery.

- Whole Foods prioritizes whole, unprocessed foods. Fruits, vegetables, lean meats, complete grains, and healthy fats should make up the majority of your diet.

- Meal Planning: Making a plan for your meals will help you ensure that you get a variety of nutrients throughout the day. This helps keep you from making rash or harmful choices.

- Consume with awareness: Recognize when you are hungry and full. By enjoying your meals and taking your time, you may prevent overeating.

- Supplements: To compensate for vitamin shortages, consider taking supplements if necessary. Consult a medical professional before adding supplements to your regimen.

- Consistency is key: Stick to a regular eating schedule to sustain your metabolism and energy levels.

- Track Your Progress: Use a food journal or a monitoring tool to track how much food you eat and how it relates to your goals.

EXERCISE PROGRAMS

Heart-Based Ignition

Exercises Using High-Intensity Interval Training (HIIT):

High-intensity interval training (HIIT), a crucial part of the Metabolic Reset Exercise program, is well known for its capacity to efficiently boost metabolism, enhance cardiovascular fitness, and improve general endurance. HIIT involves short bursts of high-intensity exercise separated by rest or low-intensity activity periods. This technique will challenge both your anaerobic and aerobic systems, which will greatly boost your physical and metabolic fitness.

Important HIIT Exercise Components:

- Brief, High-Intensity Bursts: HIIT exercises are made up of short, high-intensity bursts of activity that occur when you are almost at your maximum effort. Exercises like burpees, jumping jacks, and jogging may fall under this category.

- Recuperation Times: In between periods of high activity, there are periods of active recovery or complete rest. Recovery causes your heart rate to decrease, giving you time to catch your breath and prepare for the next difficult stage.

- Diversification: HIIT workouts may be changed to suit individuals with varying fitness levels and preferences. You may adjust the duration, intervals, and exercises to suit your ability level.

- Time Effectiveness: High-intensity interval training is well known for its efficiency. They have quicker impacts than steady-state aerobic exercises.

Overdosing on oxygen after exercise (EPOC) is an "afterburn" consequence of high-intensity interval training (HIIT). This suggests that your body keeps burning calories even after you stop exercising.

How to put together a HIIT exercise:

- Prepare yourself by warming up for five to ten minutes to activate your heart and muscles. This can involve dynamic stretching and vigorous exercise.

- Structure of Intervals: Switch off between periods of intense exertion and rest. Thirty seconds of exertion and thirty seconds of rest is the standard ratio of 1:1.

- Exercise Selection: Choose activities that challenge many muscle groups and elevate your heart rate. Some exercises include mountain climbers, kettlebell swings, jumping jacks, and sprints.

- Duration: Start with 15–20 minute workouts and gradually increase them as your level of fitness rises.

- Cool-down: After your workout, spend five to ten minutes doing static stretches and deep breathing to promote flexibility and recovery.

The advantages of HIIT workouts

- Effective Calorie Burn: High-intensity interval training (HIIT) boosts calorie burn in a shorter period, making it the ideal workout for those with busy schedules.

- Metabolic Boost: By speeding up your metabolism, HIIT enhances calorie burn even after physical activity.

- Cardiovascular Fitness: By raising your cardiovascular endurance, HIIT improves the health of your heart and lungs.

- Time Savings: HIIT allows you to achieve significant fitness gains in a shorter time than traditional cardio activities.

- Adaptability: HIIT is suitable for both beginners and specialists since it can be modified to suit individuals with different levels of fitness.

Increasing Vitality and Endurance:

Increasing your stamina and endurance is a crucial part of the metabolic reset workout regimen, which enhances your general health and fitness. While stamina refers to the power and tenacity required to endure strenuous activities, endurance is your body's ability to sustain physical activity over an extended length of time. Improving these characteristics will help you become fitter and enable you to exercise for longer periods, which will have a greater beneficial effect on your metabolism.

Among the techniques to improve stamina and endurance are:

- Cardiovascular Exercise: Engage in regular cardiovascular exercise such as brisk walking, cycling, swimming, or running. Increase the duration and intensity of your exercises progressively to put your cardiovascular system under stress.

- Interval Training: Because HIIT workouts mix short bursts of high-intensity activity with rest intervals, they are excellent for building endurance and stamina.

- Progressive Overload: Gradually increase the resistance, duration, or intensity of your workouts to foster adaptation and endurance gains.

- Long-Distance Training: By including longer steady-state cardio exercises, you may increase your body's capability for continuous exertion. Your body will be pushed to its limits by this.

- Cross-training: Mix up your exercise routines to target various muscle groups and prevent overuse injuries. Exercises that include cross-training include dance, swimming, and cycling.

- Appropriate nutrition: Consume a balanced diet to provide your body with the energy it needs for prolonged physical exercise.

- Sufficient Rest: Take enough naps and allow your body to heal in between strenuous exercise sessions. Ensure that you are receiving enough sleep and allowing your body enough time to heal.

- Breathing techniques: To optimize oxygen intake and boost endurance during exercise, use the appropriate breathing techniques.

Safely developing endurance and stamina involves:

- Advancement Slowly: By gradually increasing the duration and intensity of your workouts, you can avoid overexertion. Excessive exercise too soon might lead to burnout or accidents.

- Pay Attention to Your Body: Observe how your body adjusts to increasing pressure. If you are tired or in pain, do not push yourself to go on.

- Prioritize your recovery by following a healthy post-workout diet, drinking enough water, stretching, and getting enough rest.

- Maintaining consistency is the key to building endurance and stamina. Regularly work your heart and gradually increase the difficulty.

Power Unleashed

Compound Exercises that Engage the Whole Body:

The Metabolic Reset Exercise program relies heavily on compound exercises to maximize training efficiency and achieve whole-body gains in fitness. Compound exercises increase overall functional strength, improve muscle activation, and engage many muscle groups and joints simultaneously. They also increase calorie expenditure.

Advantages of compound workouts include:

- Effective Workouts: Compound exercises promote the development of all major muscle groups and save time by allowing you to work several muscle groups in a single action.

- Calorie Burn: Exerting more muscles requires you to expend more energy, which raises your calorie burn during and after a workout.

- Functioning Power: Compound movements, which mimic real-life activities, can enhance your capacity to do routine tasks and sports-related activities.

- Hormonal Reaction: By inducing the production of growth hormone and testosterone, compound exercises aid in the development of muscles and the removal of fat.

- Core Participation: Because it improves posture and core strength, core stability is essential for many challenging activities.

Compounds That Work Exercises:

- Squat: This exercise works the quadriceps, hamstrings, glutes, and lower back. It is an essential exercise for building strength in the lower body.

- Deadlift: A deadlift works the back, hamstrings, glutes, and core. It works wonders for building overall strength.

- Bench Press: This exercise works the triceps, shoulders, and chest. The main purpose of it is to strengthen the upper body.

- Pull-ups and chin-ups: These improve upper body pulling power by strengthening the shoulders, biceps, and upper back.

- Push-Ups: Using the chest, shoulders, triceps, and core, push-ups enhance upper-body pushing power.

- Bended-Over: Rows: This exercise improves upper body pulling power by strengthening the biceps, lats, and upper back.

- Lunges: By using the quadriceps, hamstrings, glutes, and core, lunges help to develop and stabilize the lower body.

- Overhead Press: To improve pressing power in the upper body, this exercise targets the shoulders, triceps, and upper back.

Including the compound workouts

- Balanced Routine: Include challenging exercises that focus on a variety of muscle groups in your fitness regimen.

- Compound movements may be used to create full-body workout plans that specifically target important muscle groups.

- Progressive Overload: Increasing the weight or intensity of your compound exercises progressively will promote strength gain.

- Warm-Up: Make time for a rigorous warm-up to prepare your joints and muscles for challenging activities.

- Form and Technique: To prevent mishaps, pay close attention to proper form. Consider working with a fitness professional to guarantee correct execution.

- Recovery: Take enough breaks and time to relax in between challenging workouts to prevent overtraining.

Gaining Weight and Lean Muscle:

Gaining lean muscle mass is a crucial component of the Metabolic Reset Exercise program since it improves your overall strength, speeds up your metabolism, and supports long-term health in addition to boosting your physical attractiveness. Lean muscle growth requires a balance of intentional exercise, a healthy diet, and strategic rest.

The importance of gaining muscular mass

- Metabolic Boost: The basal metabolic rate is raised by muscle tissue because it consumes more calories at rest than fat tissue.

- Better Body Composition: Increasing muscle mass while reducing body fat leads to a leaner, more defined physique.

- Strength and utility: Increased muscle mass leads to greater functional strength, which facilitates the completion of everyday tasks.

- Bone wellness: Gaining muscular mass may increase bone density and reduce the incidence of osteoporosis.

Among the methods for building lean muscle mass are:

- Resistance training: Engage in intricate movements that target the major muscle groups regularly.

- Progressive Overload: Raise the resistance or weight you lift progressively to continuously challenge your muscles and promote growth.

- Nutrition: Consume a lot of protein-rich foods to provide your muscles with the building blocks they need for growth and healing.

- Balanced Diet: To support overall health and ensure that your body has the resources it needs to gain muscle, eat a variety of high-nutrient meals.

- Eat enough calories to support muscle growth while ensuring that your caloric intake is balanced with your goals.

- Post-exercise Nutrition: Eat a meal or snack that includes both protein and carbohydrates as soon as possible after your workout to promote muscle growth and recovery.
- Rest and Recovery: Your muscles build and repair during the time they spend at rest between training sessions.

Muscle-building workouts that work well include:

- Compound Motions: Squats, deadlifts, bench presses, rows, and overhead presses are a few examples of exercises that are great for gaining muscle since they work for many muscle groups.
- Exercises using isolation: These exercises, which include leg extensions, triceps extensions, and bicep curls, target specific muscular areas.

Consistency and patience

- Consistency: Building lean muscular mass takes time. It's critical to maintain consistency in your food and workout regimen for the greatest outcomes.
- Have patience: It takes time to gain muscle. Never evaluate your progress about others'. Have patience.
- Tracking Progress: Keep track of your strength improvements and snap photos to show how things change over time.
- Make rest and sleep a priority to improve muscle growth and recuperation.

- Professional Advice: If you're new to strength training, think about working with a fitness specialist to ensure proper technique and programming.

PHASE OF PROGRESSION: ENHANCING YOUR ACHIEVEMENTS

Observing and Modifying Your Exercise Schedule

When utilizing the Metabolic Reset Exercise program, it's important to monitor and adjust your exercise plan to ensure continual growth, prevent plateaus, and adapt to your body's changing needs. Regularly paying close attention to assessment ensures that your workouts are fruitful and aligned with your goals.

It is vital to observe and make adjustments.

- Progress tracking: By monitoring your growth, you may assess your progress and identify areas in which you still have room for improvement.

- Steering Clear of Plateaus: As your body adapts, you may experience a plateau. To keep moving and avoid stagnation, your body needs to be adjusted.

- Maximizing Results: By modifying your plan as you go, you may make your workouts more effective and reach your objectives more quickly.

Procedures for Seeing and Adjusting:

- Define the assessment interval: You might decide on a weekly, bimonthly, or monthly schedule for your progress reviews.

- Monitor key metrics: Monitor key information like weight, body measurements, strength improvements, and the fit of your clothes.

- Assess Your Mood: Reflect on your sentiments both during and after your exercise. Are you becoming stronger? Have you got more energy?

- Evaluate Your Goals: Return often to your initial goals. Are you approaching them with more progress?

- Alter Depending on Progress: If you're seeing results, think about progressively increasing the complexity or intensity of your exercises. Should the progress be slower, assess the circumstances and adjust your approach.

- Plateau Administration: If you find that you are stuck, try changing the order in which you do the exercises, introducing new exercises, increasing the weight or repetitions, or modifying the rest periods.

- Provide Variability: To keep things fresh and encourage muscle growth, try introducing different workouts or routines.

- Listen to Your Body: Pay attention to the messages that your body is sending forth. If you find that you're often exhausted or in pain, it may be time to adjust your approach.
- Nutrition Analysis: Review the foods you eat. Are you giving yourself enough food to fuel your workouts? As needed, adjust.

Expert counsel

- A fitness expert: You may want to see a fitness specialist for guidance if you're not sure how to modify your approach.
- Healthcare Professional: Consult your physician before altering your exercise routine if you have any health concerns.

Keeping an Upbeat Attitude

- Remain composed: Development may not always follow a straight path. Remain composed and focus on the greater picture.
- Honor your accomplishments: No matter how little, acknowledging your accomplishments keeps you inspired.
- Remain adaptable: Things in life aren't always foreseeable. If circumstances change, be prepared to adjust your plan of action.

Monitoring Metabolic Alterations

To understand how your body responds to your efforts at exercise and food, tracking changes in your metabolism is a crucial component of the Metabolic Reset Exercise program. Monitoring key metabolic metrics can help you fine-tune your approach, accelerate your growth, and reach your desired levels of health and fitness.

Important metrics for tracking changes in metabolism

- composition of the body: first Take regular measurements of your weight, lean muscle mass, and body fat % to track any changes in your composition.
- Resting Metabolic Rate: Track your RMR regularly to find out how effectively your body utilizes energy at rest. Improved metabolic performance is indicated by an increase in RMR.
- Monitor your energy levels at all times of the day. A higher level of energy might be a sign of a better metabolism.
- Physical Performance: Track your improvements in strength, endurance, and power. Better performance often corresponds with a more sensitive metabolism.
- Hormonal Harmony: Be mindful of hormonal alterations, such as elevated insulin sensitivity and balanced cortisol levels, that may impact metabolism.

- Subjective Experience: Observe any changes in cravings, satiety, and appetite. Improved metabolism might result from positive changes.

Methods of Tracking Metabolic Alterations

- Regular assessments: Make an appointment with a certified health professional, dietitian, or fitness specialist regularly to monitor body composition and metabolic markers.

- Self-monitoring: Keep track of your workouts, food, energy levels, and overall health in a notebook. Information on changes and trends may be obtained from this.

- Monitoring Apps: Use apps for nutrition and fitness tracking to stay on top of your daily progress, meals, and activities.

- Measurements and photos: Take frequent body measurements and progress photos to visually track changes.

- Lab testing: It's important to consider comprehensive lab testing that measures the levels of metabolic markers including hormones, cholesterol, and glucose.

Recognizing and Adjusting to Change

- Good adjustments consist of: If you see improvements in your KPIs, stick to your current plan. Reliability is crucial.

- Stability or Regression: If you're not seeing the desired effects, consider making changes to your recovery, nutrition, or workout regimen.

- Expert Advice: Seek advice from professionals such as dietitians, exercise instructors, or medical professionals if you need assistance in interpreting the changes.

Using a conscious strategy.

- It takes time for metabolism to change, thus patience is a virtue. Refrain from making big changes in reaction to short-term fluctuations and exercise patience.
- A Holistic Approach: Remember that a variety of factors, including lifestyle in general, stress, sleep, and hydration, may affect metabolic health.

Adapting Your Nutritional Approach

Ensuring your dietary choices align with your evolving fitness goals and metabolic needs is a continuous effort while following the Metabolic Reset Exercise program. You may optimize your performance, enhance metabolic efficiency, and advance your overall wellness by adjusting your nutrition plan as your body responds to exercise and lifestyle modifications.

- Assess the existing action plan: Examine your current eating plan. Are you receiving enough nourishment and energy? Are you making progress toward your goals?
- Listen to Your Body: Observe how different meals make you feel physically. Do certain meals leave you feeling nauseous or low on energy?

- Evaluate Progress: Consider what you've accomplished and determine if any adjustments are necessary to keep things going ahead.

- New Goals: If you've decided to shift your fitness goals from weight loss to muscle gain, you need to adjust your food plan accordingly.

- Post-Workout Nutrition: Make sure your meals after working out include the nutrients your body needs to repair and build muscle.

- Meal Timing: Consider the time of day you eat. Frequent meals may keep your energy levels stable and prevent overindulging.

- Hydrolysis: Adequate hydration is necessary for optimal metabolic processes. Keep an eye on how much water you're drinking and adjust as needed.

- Micronutrients: A variety of vitamins and minerals from whole meals should be consumed to support overall health.

Adapting Your Dietary Scheme:

- Calorie Intake: Adjust your calorie intake based on how your level of activity, your goals, and your progress are changing. This may include modifying the calorie intake, depending on the circumstances.

- Macro Ratios: Match the ratios of your macronutrients to your current goals. For example, increasing protein intake may aid in promoting the growth of muscles.
- Healthy Eating: Give whole, nutrient-dense foods top attention. Limit your consumption of processed foods and sugar-filled beverages.
- Portion Control: Pay attention to how much you consume to avoid overindulging. If appropriate, make use of tracking tools or portion rules.
- Meal Ingredients: Make sure each meal has a combination of fiber, complex carbohydrates, protein, and healthy fats.
- Experimentation: Try out different meals and eating habits to see what suits your body and goals the best.

Keeping an Upbeat Attitude

- Have flexibility: Your diet should suit your preferences and way of life. Being flexible helps one avoid feeling constrained.
- Have patience: The results of dietary adjustments may not show up right away. The key is to exercise patience.
- Baby Steps: Avoid making big changes by starting with little, gradual steps. Modest but durable modifications are more likely to be maintained.

PHASE OF TRANSFORMATION: ACKNOWLEDGING YOUR POTENTIAL

Honoring Achievements and Milestones

Not only is it exciting to celebrate your successes and milestones when you follow the Metabolic Reset Exercise program, but it's also an important way to stay inspired, value your work, and have a positive mindset as you continue through your fitness journey. Acknowledging your successes, no matter how little, keeps you motivated and dedicated.

The importance of commemorating

- Motivational Kick: Reaching milestones fills you with a sense of accomplishment that spurs you to keep going.
- Positive reinforcement: Giving attention to your accomplishments motivates positive behaviors and habits.
- Enhanced Attention: Holidays act as a gentle reminder of your goals and the main reasons you are participating in your exercise regimen.
- Long-term perspective: By acknowledging and appreciating your little victories, you may be able to better understand your progress toward your ultimate goals.

How to Pay Tribute to Important Events and Achievements

- Establish Mini-Goals: Break down your loftier goals into smaller, celebratory benchmarks.

- Reward yourself with something unique, like new workout gear, a massage, a night out, or a relaxing day at home.

- Share with Others: Let the fitness industry and/or your social circle know about your achievements. Their compliments and words of support might be quite motivating.

- Journaling: Keep a log of your successes and personal development. Reflecting on your trip may bring you happiness.

- Social media: Post your successes on social media to let your network know you're proud of them and to encourage others.

- Reflect mindfully: Give yourself some time to recognize your accomplishments and the fruits of your labor.

Advice on Sustaining a Positive Outlook:

- Concentrate on Progress: Acknowledge the journey and remember that every step you take will get you one step closer to your goals.

- Accept setbacks: Rather than seeing them as failures, view them as lessons learned. Continue to maintain your flexibility.

- Avoid comparing your progress to that of others by practicing comparison awareness. Everybody's journey is distinct, and each person advances at a different rate.
- Gratitude: Learn to be grateful for your physical gifts, your labors, and the progress you've made.

Fostering sustained success

- Rewarding yourself for your accomplishments regularly creates a positive feedback loop that encourages perseverance.
- Factors that Drive Motivation From Within: Take pride in your achievements for their own sake as well as the advantages they will have beyond the home.
- Mind-Body Relationship: Acknowledge that the positive changes your body and mind are experiencing are a direct result of your efforts.

Techniques for Breaking Through Plateaus

Reaching plateaus in the metabolic reset exercise program is a common occurrence. If you have the right mindset and strategy, however, you can get beyond these periods of inertia and continue working toward your goals. Plateaus provide opportunities for growth, flexibility, and technique enhancement.

How to Interpret A Plateau

- Normal Phase: Plateauing is a common occurrence in any fitness program. Your progress may temporarily stop while your body adjusts to your routine.

- Period: Plateaus may happen within a few weeks or months. Be patient and tenacious.

- Change your mindset such that plateaus are seen as opportunities to refine your approach rather than as signs of failure.

Methods for Overcoming a Plateau:

- Change Up Your Routine: Add diversity by altering your sessions, raising the weights, or trying other training approaches.

- Modify the difficulty of your workouts by adding more reps, bigger weights, or longer rest intervals.

- Switch to a New Program: Alter your exercise regimen to shock your muscles and trigger fresh energy sources.

- Nutritional Adjustments: Evaluate your approach to eating. Are you consuming the right nutrients in the right proportions to help you achieve your goals?

- Periodization: Make sure to include periodization, which involves alternating between sessions of high and low intensity.

- Rest & Recuperation: Be careful to provide enough time for self-care during the intervals between sessions. Overtraining may impede peak performance.

- Focus on Weak Points: Identify your body's weakest muscle groups to help you maintain equilibrium.

- Mindful Consumption: Be mindful of the amount you consume and the way you eat to ensure that your body is receiving the finest nourishment available.

- Sleep Quality: Make sleep a priority since not getting enough sleep might hinder your progress.

Staying positive and patient:

- Change Your Attitude: See plateaus as temporary setbacks rather than unachievable barriers.

- Examine your progress by going over your previous achievements. There are plateaus along the way.

- Honor non-scale victories: Even if the scale isn't moving, acknowledge improvements in strength, stamina, and overall health.

- Establish Micro-Goals: Pay attention to little goals that you can achieve when you're at a standstill.

- Practice mindfulness and meditation to reduce stress and keep your mental toughness.

Expert counsel

- Speak with experts: If you're unsure of how to break through a plateau, obtain guidance from dietitians, fitness instructors, or healthcare professionals.

- Adjust Gradually: Make incremental adjustments to prevent abrupt, painful changes.

Changing Course and Proceeding:

- Look at this as an opportunity to learn: plateaus teach you about your body's responses and make you more adaptable.

- Remain Committed: When you hit a plateau in your fitness regimen, it's important to keep up your commitment to it.

Living the Lifestyle of a Metabolic Reset

Taking up the metabolic reset lifestyle means embracing a holistic approach to health that includes self-care, self-feeding, mental health, and exercise. It extends beyond food and exercise. Taking up this lifestyle will not only help you look better, but it will also help you form long-lasting habits that will improve your overall health.

The following are the main elements of the metabolic reset lifestyle:

- Physical Activity: Strength training, high-intensity interval training, and cardiovascular exercises should all be a part of your everyday regimen.

- Nutrition: Give your body full, nutrient-dense meals to support healthy energy levels, muscle growth, and overall well-being.

- Motivation: Develop a resilient, upbeat mindset that will help you overcome setbacks, celebrate your successes, and maintain your motivation.

- Rest and Recovery: Prioritize getting adequate sleep, control your stress, and give your body time to recover from activity.

- Hydration: To support a healthy metabolism and overall wellness, make sure you drink enough water throughout the day.

- Mindful Eating: Practice mindful eating to prevent overeating and to foster a healthy relationship with food.

- Self-Care: Incorporate self-care practices such as relaxation techniques, meditation, and engaging in hobbies that enhance your mental and emotional health.

- Be consistent in your lifestyle decisions to create long-lasting habits that help you achieve your goals.

Adopting a Lifestyle of Metabolic Reset:

- Establish Intentions: State your objectives and plans for adopting the metabolic reset lifestyle to establish your intentions. What are you hoping to achieve? In what way would you want to feel?

- Establish a Routine: Make a daily plan that includes meals, exercise, and self-care activities.

- Plan: Make your meals, schedule exercise, and schedule restorative activities to maintain a balanced lifestyle.

- Honor Progress: Draw attention to both little and large achievements. Honoring your accomplishments encourages positive behavior.

- Mindful Choices: Whether it's selecting a nutritious meal or prioritizing exercise, make thoughtful choices that help you achieve your goals.

- Exercise Patience: Remember that committing to a metabolic reset lifestyle takes time and effort. It takes time to find things.

- Adapt and Evolve: Be prepared to adjust your plan in response to new requirements, evolving goals, and personal growth.

Bringing about permanent change

- The comprehensive change: Adopting a metabolic reset lifestyle entails more than just making physical changes. It is about whole health—that is, the state of one's body, mind, and soul.

- Long-Term Wellness: By choosing this lifestyle, you are investing in your long-term well-being and vitality.

- Continuing education: To refine your approach, maintain an open mind, and keep learning about wellness in general, exercise, and diet.

- Motivating Others: By leading the Metabolic Reset lifestyle, you set an example for others around you and encourage them to go on their journeys.

MAINTAINING YOUR ACHIEVEMENT

Consistency and Long-Term Upkeep

The benefits of the Metabolic Reset Exercise program must be sustained over time with a commitment to adaptability, consistency, and a sustainable mindset toward exercise, food, and overall health. By adopting balanced thinking and integrating healthful behaviors into your daily routine, you may ensure sustained success and continuous progress.

Long-term maintenance techniques include:

- Establish achievable long-term objectives that will act as a roadmap and motivation for your journey. These should be realistic ambitions.

- Adopt a Lifestyle: Shift your perspective to one of a lifelong dedication to health and wellness rather than one of short fixes.

- The secret is consistency: You should stick to your routine of regular exercise and a nutritious diet even after you've reached your initial goals.

- Frequent Check-Ins: Keep track of your progress, adjust your goals, and change your plan of action as needed by doing frequent check-ins.

- Variation: Keep your workouts fresh to prevent boredom and to guarantee ongoing physical development.

- Mindful Eating: Continue to practice mindful eating to have a healthy relationship with food and prevent overindulging.

- Self-Care: To enhance general wellness, give priority to stress reduction techniques, peaceful sleep, and relaxation techniques.

- Keep Moving: Whether you like dance, hiking, or sports, discover joy in movement by engaging in your passions.

- Professional Advice: Seek advice from medical professionals or fitness specialists for ongoing guidance and adjustments.

Acclimating to Shifts

- First Life Transitions: Be prepared to modify your plan when travel, job changes, or family duties cause you to miss scheduled time.

- Aging: Your body's needs and responses change as you age. Modify your routine to account for your changing physiology.

- Reversals: If you encounter difficulties, consider them temporary impediments rather than justifications for giving up.

Drive and disposition:

- Internal Motivation: Enjoy the process of self-care, which leads to the development of intrinsic motivation.
- Celebrate Your Progress: Keep appreciating your accomplishments and landmarks, no matter where you are in your journey.
- Positive Self-Talk: To increase your dedication to long-term wellness, replace negative self-affirmations with positive ones.

Establishing a Cozy Ambience

- Embrace your surroundings by joining a community of supportive individuals who share your goals for your physical and mental well-being.
- Family and Friends: To positively influence them at home, encourage your loved ones to adopt healthy habits alongside you.

Thinking back and being thankful:

- Practice Gratitude: Consistently reflect on the benefits of leading a healthy lifestyle and the advantageous adjustments you've made.
- Studying and Growth: Continue learning about fitness, nutrition, and health to enhance your approach and keep participants interested.

"Resilient Success" denotes:

- Strive for progress rather than perfection and accept imperfection. In the long run, consistency matters more than mistakes in judgment.

- Life-Long Road: Acknowledge that you will always have new goals and challenges to achieve on your journey to health and happiness.

- Make self-compassion and self-care a priority, knowing that this will enhance every aspect of your life.

Including Metabolic Reset in Everyday Activities

You may incorporate the Metabolic Reset Exercise program into your daily life by making conscious choices that prioritize your fitness goals, overall health, and well-being. With seamless integration of the program's principles into your everyday activities, you may create a long-lasting lifestyle that supports success and vitality.

Techniques for Daily Integration:

- Morning routine: Start your day with a few minutes of stretching, deep breathing, or quick exercise to boost your energy and metabolism.

- Meal Planning: To avoid making poor food choices at the last minute, be sure to plan balanced meals and snacks.

- Active Commute: If at all possible, try to cycle or walk to work to maintain an active lifestyle throughout the day.

- Workouts for the lunch break: Use your lunch hour to engage in a little workout, whether it's a rapid yoga session, bodyweight exercises, or a brisk walk.

- If you want to increase your daily activity level and speed up your metabolism, use the stairs rather than the elevator.

- Hydration Reminder: To improve your metabolic processes and stay hydrated, set reminders to drink water throughout the day.

- Snack Wisely: Opt for nutrient-dense snacks like fruits, nuts, and yogurt to keep your energy levels constant.

- Desk stretches: Perform simple stretches and movements at your workspace to improve circulation and prevent stiffness.

- Exercise in the Evening: Perform a vigorous workout or a contemplative yoga session in the evening to help you relax and promote healing.

Creating a friendly atmosphere

- To make it simpler to work out often, set up a room in your home for this purpose.

- Organize your pantry with wholesome foods that go well with the metabolic reset plan.

- Locate an "Accountability Partner" who shares your goals for physical fitness. This individual is going to be an inspiration to you both.
- Remove temptations: Keep unhealthy foods hidden to avoid impulsive munching.

Applying mindfulness

- Employ a range of strategies: Vary your routines and attempt new workouts to prevent boredom.
- Savor the Journey: Pay attention to the beneficial shifts you experience as you accept the process of adopting a healthier lifestyle.

Flexibility and Adaptability:

- Listen to Your Body: Pay attention to the signals coming from your body, and adjust your routine based on how you're feeling.
- Life Happens: Accept that some days could be busier than others and that it's OK to adjust your schedule as needed.

Tracking of progress

- Journaling: Keep a fitness journal where you may document your workouts, food, and progress overall.
- To visually track your development, measure and take pictures of your progress regularly.

Self-care and meditation:

- Mindful Eating: Savor each bite of food while paying attention to your body's signals of hunger and fullness.

- Techniques for Relaxation: Make time for techniques for relaxation such as gentle stretching, deep breathing, or meditation.

An extended perspective is:

- Consistent Habits: You will progressively incorporate the Metabolic Reset program into your daily activities.

- Adopt the program as a lifelong commitment to health and well-being—a lifestyle, not a phase.

Motivating Others: Expressing Your Experience

As you complete the Metabolic Reset Exercise program and see changes in your health and wellness, sharing your story may inspire and motivate others to begin their paths to fitness and vitality. Your triumphs, setbacks, and life lessons may serve as an inspiration to others who want to make significant changes.

Successful Methods for Inspiring People:

- Authenticity: Talk about your journey with sincerity. People engage when you use relatable experiences and real-world examples.

- Give a brief explanation of your motivation for starting the program and how it aligns with your goals and values.

- Progress updates consist of Regularly updating your loved ones or followers on social media on your progress, emphasizing both little and big victories.

- Before and after: Changes in appearance might serve as powerful motivators. Add pictures of the before and after to your story.

- Problems and Suggestions: What difficulties did you run across, and how did you resolve them? This shows that while there are challenges along the path, they can be surmounted.

- Advice and Methods: Talk about healthy eating habits, weight-loss strategies, and methods that you have found effective.

- Motivation and Mindset: Talk about the emotional and psychological aspects of your journey, such as how you manage to stay upbeat and motivated.

- Interact and React: Take part in the discourse with your viewers by responding to their messages and remarks.

- Empowerment: Talk about how you've taken responsibility for your journey to encourage others to do the same for their health and happiness.

Having a positive effect

- Giving an example: People may learn from your commitment and reliability.
- Offer assistance: Make yourself accessible to offer guidance and motivation to those who want counsel.
- Honor Others: Show the same gratitude for their achievements as you do for your own. Create a friendly neighborhood.

Online resources and social media platforms:

- Employ hashtags to expand your audience. Add relevant hashtags related to health and fitness.
- Share quick training videos or clips that show your dedication and progress.
- Participate in competitions. Participate in online fitness programs or challenges to connect with others pursuing similar goals.

Individual support

- Family and Friends: Share your experience with them to inspire them to join you on your search for better health.
- Local Community: Consider organizing health or fitness events in your community to inspire others and build connections.

Constructive dialogue

- Remain Upbeat: Try not to focus on the challenges you face and instead acknowledge the positive aspects of your journey.

- "Inspire, Don't Compare. You are unique on your journey." is a mantra that may be used to uplift individuals without making them feel inferior.

Respectful Sharing

- Privacy: Protect your personal space and private information; only divulge information about which you feel comfortable.

- No Obligation: Regarding their choices, bear in mind that not everyone will be ready for or interested in embarking on a fitness journey.

A 7-WEEK METABOLIC RESET EXERCISE PROGRAM SCHEDULE FOR WOMEN

I've put together a workout plan to help kickstart your metabolism. Remember, it's crucial to talk to a healthcare professional before diving into any new exercise routine, especially if you have existing health conditions. This plan includes a mix of cardio, strength training, and flexibility exercises to give you a comprehensive fitness boost.

Week 1: Cardiovascular Foundation

Day 1-3:

- Morning: 20 minutes of brisk walking or jogging
- Afternoon/Evening: Bodyweight exercises (squats, lunges, push-ups) – 3 sets of 10-15 reps each
- Flexibility: 10 minutes of stretching

Day 4: Rest or Active Recovery

- Gentle activities like yoga or walking

Day 5-7:

- Morning: 25 minutes of interval running or cycling
- Afternoon/Evening: Full-body resistance training with light weights – 3 sets of 10-12 reps each
- Flexibility: 10 minutes of yoga

Week 2: Intensity Build-Up

Day 1-3:

- Morning: 25 minutes of high-intensity interval training (HIIT)
- Afternoon/Evening: Strength training focusing on major muscle groups – 3 sets of 12-15 reps each
- Flexibility: 15 minutes of dynamic stretching

Day 4: Rest or Active Recovery

- Consider low-impact activities like swimming or cycling

Day 5-7:

- Morning: 30 minutes of cardio (running, cycling, or dance)
- Afternoon/Evening: Core workout – planks, Russian twists, leg raises – 3 sets of 12-15 reps each
- Flexibility: 15 minutes of Pilates

Week 3: Variety and Challenge

Day 1-3:

- Morning: 30 minutes of cardio (choose a different activity than Week 2)
- Afternoon/Evening: Circuit training with a mix of bodyweight and dumbbell exercises – 4 sets of 12-15 reps each
- Flexibility: 15 minutes of dynamic stretches

Day 4: Rest or Active Recovery

- Engage in activities like hiking or leisurely biking

Day 5-7:

- Morning: 35 minutes of steady-state cardio (power walking, cycling)
- Afternoon/Evening: Leg-focused workout – squats, lunges, deadlifts – 3 sets of 12-15 reps each
- Flexibility: 15 minutes of yoga

Week 4: Peak Intensity and Relaxation

Day 1-3:

- Morning: 30 minutes of HIIT
- Afternoon/Evening: Full-body strength training with increased resistance – 4 sets of 10-12 reps each
- Flexibility: 15 minutes of Pilates

Day 4: Rest or Active Recovery

- Rest or engage in gentle activities like swimming or walking

Day 5-7:

- Morning: 40 minutes of cardio (choose a favorite activity)
- Afternoon/Evening: Full-body circuit incorporating cardio and strength exercises – 4 sets of 10-15 reps each
- Flexibility: 15 minutes of relaxation yoga

Week 5: Full-Body Strength and Cardio Integration

This schedule focuses on full-body strength training and cardiovascular workouts.

Day 1: Full-Body Strength

- Squats, Push-Ups, Bent-Over Rows, Lunges and Plank

Day 2: Cardio and Core

- a 20-minute HIIT exercise (alternating between high-intensity exercises and rest periods)
- Exercises for the abdomen: crunches, leg lifts, and bicycle crunches

Day 3: Rest or Active Recovery

- Light stretching, Yoga, and A leisurely walk

Day 4: Upper Body Strength

- Bench Press, Pull-ups or late pulldowns, Overhead Shoulder Presses, Triceps dips, and Bicep Curls

Day 5: Cardio and Lower Body

- 30 minutes of moderate-intensity cardio (running, cycling, swimming), Squat Jumps, Step-Ups and Glute Bridges

Day 6: Active Recovery

- Gentle yoga, Foam rolling, or a relaxed walk.

Day 7: Rest

Week 6: Split Routine with Emphasis on Muscle Groups

With this regimen, various days are dedicated to working on different muscle groups:

Day 1: Upper Body Push

- Bench Presses, shoulder presses, Push-Ups, and Triceps Extensions

Day 2: Lower Body

- Squats, Deadlifts, Lunges, Leg curls

Day 3: Rest or Active Recovery

Day 4: Upper Body Pull

- Pull-Ups or Rows, Bent-Over Rows, Bicep Curls, Face Pulls

Day 5: HIIT Cardio

- 20-minute high-intensity interval training (HIIT) session

Day 6: Active Recovery

- Stretching, light yoga, or a leisurely walk

Day 7: Rest

Week 7: Full-Body Circuit Training

This program uses a circuit approach to blend cardiovascular and strength training.

Day 1: Circuit Training

- Perform each exercise for 30 seconds, with a 15-second rest between exercises. Complete 3–4 rounds.
- Jumping Jacks, Bodyweight Squats, Push-Ups, Plank, high knees, Bicycle crunches

Day 2: Rest or Active Recovery

Day 3: Circuit Training

- Same format as Day 1, but with different exercises:
- Burpees, Lunges, Dips, Mountain Climbers, Skaters, Russian Twists

Day 4: Cardio

- 40 minutes of moderate-intensity cardio (running, cycling, swimming)

Day 5: Active Recovery

- Light stretching, Yoga, A leisurely walk

Day 6: Rest

Day 7: Full-Body Strength

- Squats, Bench Press, Rows, Plank, and Bicep Curls

Nutritional Guidelines and Meal Plans

Nutritional Guidelines:

- ***Balanced Macronutrients:*** Try to have a meal that is composed equally of healthy fats, protein, and carbs.
- ***Whole Foods:*** Give whole, unprocessed foods high in vitamins, fiber, and minerals priority.
- ***Protein Intake:*** To assist the development and recuperation of your muscles, eat enough protein.
- ***Hydration:*** To maintain your fluids and assist your metabolism, sip plenty of water throughout the day.
- ***Portion Control:*** Pay attention to serving sizes to prevent overindulging.
- ***Regular Meals:*** To keep your energy levels stable, try to eat three major meals and one or two nutritious snacks each day.

30 Day Meal Plan:

This meal plan is designed to support your fitness journey with a variety of nutrient-dense options. Remember to pair it with regular exercise, stay hydrated, and listen to your body's signals for optimal results.

Meal Plan 1: Balanced Macros

Day 1:

- Breakfast: Scrambled eggs with spinach and whole-grain toast
- Snack: Greek yogurt with mixed berries
- Lunch: Grilled chicken breast with quinoa and roasted vegetables
- Snack: Carrot and cucumber sticks with hummus
- Dinner: Baked salmon with sweet potato and steamed broccoli

Day 2:

- Breakfast: Oatmeal with sliced banana and a sprinkle of chia seeds
- Snack: Handful of almonds and an apple
- Lunch: Turkey and avocado wrap with whole-grain tortilla
- Snack: Greek yogurt with honey and walnuts
- Dinner: Stir-fried tofu with brown rice and mixed vegetables

Day 3:

- Breakfast: Whole-grain pancakes with berries and a dollop of Greek yogurt
- Snack: Cottage cheese with pineapple chunks
- Lunch: Lentil soup with a side of whole-grain roll
- Snack: Mixed nuts and dried fruit
- Dinner: Grilled shrimp with quinoa and roasted Brussels sprouts

Day 4:

- Breakfast: Protein smoothie with almond milk, banana, and spinach
- Snack: Hard-boiled eggs with a pinch of salt
- Lunch: Quinoa bowl with black beans, corn, avocado, and salsa
- Snack: Sliced apple with almond butter
- Dinner: Baked cod with quinoa and asparagus

Day 5:

- Breakfast: Greek yogurt parfait with granola and mixed berries
- Snack: Cottage cheese with sliced peaches
- Lunch: Chicken and vegetable stir-fry with brown rice
- Snack: Trail mix with nuts and dried fruit
- Dinner: Beef and broccoli stir-fry with quinoa

Day 6:

- Breakfast: Scrambled egg whites with tomatoes, spinach, and feta cheese
- Snack: Protein bar and a small piece of dark chocolate
- Lunch: Shrimp and avocado salad with a balsamic vinaigrette dressing
- Snack: Sliced pear with cheese
- Dinner: Turkey meatballs with whole-grain spaghetti and marinara sauce

Day 7:

- Breakfast: Smoothie bowl with protein powder, banana, and mixed berries
- Snack: Hard-boiled eggs with a sprinkle of black pepper
- Lunch: Quinoa salad with grilled chicken, cherry tomatoes, and feta cheese
- Snack: Greek yogurt with a drizzle of honey
- Dinner: Grilled salmon with quinoa and roasted green beans

Meal Plan 2: Plant-Based

Day 8:

- Breakfast: Avocado toast on whole-grain bread with cherry tomatoes
- Snack: Mixed berries and a handful of nuts
- Lunch: Chickpea and vegetable curry with brown rice

- Snack: Hummus with carrot and cucumber sticks
- Dinner: Grilled portobello mushrooms with quinoa and steamed broccoli

Day 9:

- Breakfast: Chia seed pudding with almond milk and fresh fruit
- Snack: Sliced apple with peanut butter
- Lunch: Lentil and vegetable wrap with whole-grain tortilla
- Snack: Vegan protein smoothie with spinach, banana, and almond milk
- Dinner: Stuffed bell peppers with quinoa and black beans

Day 10:

- Breakfast: Vegan protein pancakes with berries and maple syrup
- Snack: Guacamole with whole-grain tortilla chips
- Lunch: Quinoa and black bean bowl with avocado
- Snack: Vegan yogurt with granola
- Dinner: Stir-fried tempeh with brown rice and mixed vegetables

Day 11:

- Breakfast: Acai bowl with coconut flakes and mixed fruit
- Snack: Raw nuts and dried fruits

- Lunch: Vegan sushi rolls with brown rice, avocado, and veggies
- Snack: Hummus with cucumber slices
- Dinner: Roasted vegetable and quinoa-stuffed bell peppers

Day 12:

- Breakfast: Vegan smoothie with kale, banana, and almond milk
- Snack: Rice cakes with almond butter
- Lunch: Chickpea and quinoa salad with a lemon-tahini dressing
- Snack: Fresh fruit salad
- Dinner: Lentil and vegetable curry with basmati rice

Day 13:

- Breakfast: Vegan protein waffles with mixed berries
- Snack: Homemade energy balls with nuts and dates
- Lunch: Sweet potato and black bean burrito bowl
- Snack: Sliced mango with lime juice
- Dinner: Grilled tofu skewers with quinoa and grilled vegetables

Day 14:

- Breakfast: Vegan breakfast burrito with tofu scramble
- Snack: Guacamole with carrot sticks

- Lunch: Spinach and mushroom vegan omelet
- Snack: Vegan yogurt parfait with granola
- Dinner: Vegan stir-fried noodles with tofu and mixed vegetables

Day 15:

- Breakfast: Chia seed pudding with almond milk and fresh fruit
- Snack: Sliced apple with peanut butter
- Lunch: Lentil and vegetable wrap with whole-grain tortilla
- Snack: Vegan protein smoothie with spinach, banana, and almond milk
- Dinner: Stuffed bell peppers with quinoa and black beans

Day 16:

- Breakfast: Vegan protein pancakes with berries and maple syrup
- Snack: Guacamole with whole-grain tortilla chips
- Lunch: Quinoa and black bean bowl with avocado
- Snack: Vegan yogurt with granola
- Dinner: Stir-fried tempeh with brown rice and mixed vegetables

Day 17:

- Breakfast: Acai bowl with coconut flakes and mixed fruit
- Snack: Raw nuts and dried fruits

- Lunch: Vegan sushi rolls with brown rice, avocado, and veggies
- Snack: Hummus with cucumber slices
- Dinner: Roasted vegetable and quinoa-stuffed bell peppers

Day 18:

- Breakfast: Vegan smoothie with kale, banana, and almond milk
- Snack: Rice cakes with almond butter
- Lunch: Chickpea and quinoa salad with a lemon-tahini dressing
- Snack: Fresh fruit salad
- Dinner: Grilled tofu skewers with quinoa and grilled vegetables

Day 19:

- Breakfast: Vegan breakfast burrito with tofu scramble
- Snack: Guacamole with carrot sticks
- Lunch: Spinach and mushroom vegan omelet
- Snack: Vegan yogurt parfait with granola
- Dinner: Vegan stir-fried noodles with tofu and mixed vegetables

Day 20:

- Breakfast: Vegan protein waffles with mixed berries
- Snack: Homemade energy balls with nuts and dates

- Lunch: Sweet potato and black bean burrito bowl
- Snack: Sliced mango with lime juice
- Dinner: Grilled portobello mushrooms with quinoa and steamed broccoli

Day 21:

- Breakfast: Avocado toast on whole-grain bread with cherry tomatoes
- Snack: Mixed berries and a handful of nuts
- Lunch: Chickpea and vegetable curry with brown rice
- Snack: Hummus with carrot and cucumber sticks
- Dinner: Grilled vegetable and quinoa-stuffed bell peppers

Meal Plan 3: High-Protein

Day 22:

- Breakfast: Scrambled eggs with smoked salmon and whole-grain toast
- Snack: Cottage cheese with pineapple chunks
- Lunch: Grilled chicken Caesar salad with lots of veggies
- Snack: Protein smoothie with banana and almond milk
- Dinner: Baked cod with quinoa and asparagus

Day 23:

- Breakfast: High-protein Greek yogurt with mixed berries
- Snack: Hard-boiled eggs with a pinch of salt

- Lunch: Turkey and avocado wrap with whole-grain tortilla
- Snack: Mixed nuts and dried fruit
- Dinner: Beef and broccoli stir-fry with quinoa

Day 24:

- Breakfast: Protein smoothie bowl with granola and sliced banana
- Snack: Low-fat cottage cheese with sliced peaches
- Lunch: Chicken and vegetable stir-fry with brown rice
- Snack: Trail mix with nuts and dried fruit
- Dinner: Turkey meatballs with whole-grain spaghetti and marinara sauce

Day 25:

- Breakfast: Omelet with spinach, tomatoes, and feta cheese
- Snack: Protein bar and a small piece of dark chocolate
- Lunch: Shrimp and avocado salad with a balsamic vinaigrette dressing
- Snack: Sliced pear with cheese
- Dinner: Grilled salmon with quinoa and roasted green beans

Day 26:

- Breakfast: High-protein smoothie with almond milk, protein powder, and berries
- Snack: Greek yogurt with honey and walnuts

- Lunch: Lentil soup with a side of whole-grain roll

- Snack: Carrot and cucumber sticks with hummus

- Dinner: Baked chicken breast with sweet potato and steamed broccoli

Day 27:

- Breakfast: Protein pancakes with mixed berries and a drizzle of maple syrup

- Snack: Cottage cheese with sliced pineapple

- Lunch: Quinoa salad with grilled chicken, cherry tomatoes, and feta cheese

- Snack: Sliced apple with almond butter

- Dinner: Grilled shrimp with quinoa and roasted Brussels sprouts

Day 28:

- Breakfast: High-protein smoothie with spinach, banana, and almond milk

- Snack: Hard-boiled eggs with a sprinkle of black pepper

- Lunch: Quinoa bowl with black beans, corn, avocado, and salsa

- Snack: Greek yogurt with a drizzle of honey

- Dinner: Baked cod with quinoa and asparagus

Day 29:

- Breakfast: Scrambled eggs with smoked salmon and whole-grain toast
- Snack: Cottage cheese with pineapple chunks
- Lunch: Grilled chicken Caesar salad with lots of veggies
- Snack: Protein smoothie with banana and almond milk
- Dinner: Baked cod with quinoa and asparagus

Day 30:

- Breakfast: High-protein Greek yogurt with mixed berries
- Snack: Hard-boiled eggs with a pinch of salt
- Lunch: Turkey and avocado wrap with whole-grain tortilla
- Snack: Mixed nuts and dried fruit
- Dinner: Beef and broccoli stir-fry with quinoa

Conclusion

The Metabolic Reset Exercise Program is a complete and revolutionary method for reaching your fitness objectives while promoting overall well-being in the world of health and wellness. We've discussed the many components of this program throughout our talk, from establishing individual fitness objectives and comprehending metabolic evaluation to creating efficient training schedules, adopting a balanced diet, and maintaining long-term consistency.

The Metabolic Reset Exercise Program is fundamentally committed to feeding your body, fortifying your mind, and fostering your soul. It goes beyond only physical alterations. In addition to modifying your physical appearance, you can cultivate lifetime habits that exude energy and pleasure by combining the power of well-designed workout routines, mindful eating, and a resilient attitude.

This journey starts with a clear grasp of your fitness objectives, which will enable you to customize your training routine to meet your goals. A comprehensive fitness program includes a variety of exercise modalities, such as compound motions for full-body involvement, HIIT (high-intensity interval training), and strength training. A well-rounded strategy that addresses many areas of fitness is ensured by balancing these factors, fostering growth, and avoiding plateaus.

The crucial part of fueling your body with the correct nutrients is supporting your exercises. You can give your metabolism the fuel it needs to function at its best, fuel your workouts, and advance your general health by developing a nutrition plan that puts a priority on balanced macronutrients, nutritious foods, and mindful eating habits. By adjusting and improving your nutrition strategy as you go through this program, you can make sure that it keeps up with your changing demands.

However, the Metabolic Reset Exercise program goes beyond the physical, highlighting the value of a good outlook, honoring achievements, and encouraging self-care routines. You can overcome obstacles, stay motivated, and enjoy the nuances of the trip by developing a robust mental attitude. The skill of marking occasions and accomplishments adds a layer of motivation that strengthens your commitment, turning each step forward into a triumph to be treasured.

The real change happens when you go from a program to a lifestyle. By incorporating the metabolic reset principles into your daily routine, you can effortlessly balance your exercise, diet, rest, and self-care, building a solid foundation for your long-term well-being. This way of living respects the ebb and flow of life's demands while ensuring that your health always comes first. It celebrates variety, flexibility, and adaptation.

Keep in mind that your journey is not taking place in solitude as you go ahead. By disclosing your struggles, victories, and lessons learned, you serve as an example for others who are looking for their route to health. You are a living example of the metabolic reset concept and a monument to the strength of dedication, perseverance, and resolve.

The Metabolic Reset Exercise Program is a dynamic, changing adventure that represents your individuality and ambitions; it is not a one-size-fits-all formula. You are shaping not just your physical appearance but also the narrative of your personal health story when you establish your first objectives and adopt a lifestyle of vitality. Remember that every decision you make, every exercise you do, and every nutritional meal you eat contribute to a life filled with power, joy, and permanent health as you set out on this changing path.